THE HORMONE
natural healing
cookbook

Recipes to lose weight, re-balance & reset your metabolism.
The hormone fix & cure.

THE HORMONE NATURAL HEALING COOKBOOK

RECIPES TO LOSE WEIGHT, RE-BALANCE & RESET YOUR METABOLISM. THE HORMONE FIX & CURE.

ISBN: 978-1-913174-05-7

DISCLAIMER

CONTENTS

DINNER RECIPES

SNACKS, SWEET TREATS AND SIDE DISHES   **77**

INTRODUCTION

By using the recipes in this book, alongside intermittent fasting for the first 10 days, you will be able to kick start your system into producing new hormone receptors and speed up your metabolic rate. Your hormone levels will become stabilised and you will be relieved of metabolic stall and weight gain, hot flushes, night sweats, insomnia, memory loss or brain fog, irritability, low libido, and painful sex.

WHERE DOES IT COME FROM?

Throughout their lives, women are told that various health problems they may experience, including bad skin, mood swings, changes in libido and weight gain, are all affected by 'hormones'. But for a term that is so commonly used, it is widely misunderstood.

WHAT ARE HORMONES?

People often think of hormones in terms of the sex hormones - oestrogen, progesterone and testosterone. However, the human body produces many different types of hormone in its endocrine system. These hormones are produced in glands found all over the body and have lots of different roles to play. The main ones are:

Pituitary: The pituitary gland makes the hormones that trigger growth.
Hypothalamus: The hypothalamus gland is responsible for regulating body temperature, hunger, moods and the release of hormones from other glands. It also controls thirst, sleep and sex drive.
Parathyroid: This gland controls the amount of calcium found in the body.
Thymus: This gland plays a role in the function of the immune system and produces T-cells.
Pancreas: This gland produces the insulin that helps control blood sugar levels.
Thyroid: The thyroid produces hormones associated with calorie burning and heart rate.
Adrenal: Adrenal glands produce the hormones that control sex drive and cortisol, the stress hormone.
Pineal: Also called the thalamus, this gland produces serotonin derivatives of melatonin, which affects sleep.
Ovaries: Only found in women, the ovaries secrete oestrogen and progesterone, the female sex hormones, as well as, testosterone.
Testes: Only found in men, the testes produce the male sex hormone, testosterone, and produce sperm.

these hormones, it is surprisingly not the sex hormones that have the biggest part to play in women's day to y well-being. Instead its cortisol – the stress hormone, insulin – which regulates blood sugar, and oxytocin – metimes known as 'the love hormone', which need to be balanced in order for us to feel healthy.

WHAT HAPPENS WHEN YOUR HORMONES ARE IMBALANCED?

Hormone levels fluctuate throughout our lives to accommodate ageing. This is a natural process that allows us to grow, reach sexual maturity and bear children. In our younger years, our growth hormones are at their highest levels as we reach our adult height and hormones begin to be produced each month by our pituitary glands. This allows us to release eggs and menstruate. As we enter our twenties, our bone density reaches its peak, alongside fertility. In our thirties, the metabolism begins to slow down, but our sex hormones are still at their highest, meaning that women's libidos are high during peak years of fertility.

As we reach our forties, we see our bodies enter the perimenopause (the period before menopause), where oestrogen and progesterone levels drop, and fertility decreases. With this, you may experience a number of issues including missed periods, PMS, breakthrough bleeding, palpitations, migraines, hot flushes, vaginal dryness, insomnia and anxiety.

After this, women reach menopause. Contrary to popular belief, this is not the time when your period stops, but rather twelve months after your last period. The average age for this is 51. Some women may be lucky enough to experience very few side effects, but for many it's a time when a reduction in oestrogen results in hair loss, ache aches and pains, fatigue and weight gain – particularly on the stomach, thighs, buttocks and chin.

As we get into the post-menopausal stage, women often find that changes to the vagina occur, which can make sex uncomfortable or even painful, while skin becomes thinner, hair turns grey and they begin to lose skeletal calcium and bone mass.

All of this makes for very depressing reading, but it is a natural part of life. However, this does not have to mean that the side effects of menopause and ageing cannot be alleviated. By eating well, the likelihood of metabolic stall and weight gain, hot flushes, night sweats, insomnia, memory loss or brain fog, irritability, low libido, and painful sex, can all be reduced.

In order to understand how to do this, we must go back to look at the key hormones; insulin, cortisol and oxytocin, to see how we can use our diet to better regulate them.

HORMONES AND DIET

By adopting a ketogenic (high fat and low carb) diet, alongside lifestyle changes that bring your body's PH (power of hydrogen) levels down to a healthy alkaline level, you are able to reduce hormone resistance, leading to weight loss and increased energy levels.

Studies have shown that by reducing your urine's PH levels you can alleviate the negative symptoms discussed above. Foods that have high mineral content, such as fruits and vegetables, are the most alkaline. Meat, poultry, dairy, sugar, processed foods, grains, and caffeine are all acidic. When you eat a highly acidic diet, minerals like magnesium, calcium, potassium and bicarbonate become low, which adversely impacts your health.

Studies have shown that a diet that is high in alkaline food results in:

· **Improved bone health**
· **Lean muscle mass**
· **Optimised magnesium levels**
· **Reduced pain and inflammation**
· **Reduced risk of cardiovascular disease, cancer, and other chronic diseases**

Studies have shown that a ketogenic diet has multiple health benefits including:

- Weight loss
- Slower ageing
- A reduction in polycystic ovary syndrome (PCOS) symptoms
- Reduced acne
- Reduction in neurological issues such as Alzheimer's disease and Parkinson's disease, and reduced levels of cancer, depression and diabetes
- Increased energy levels

However, acidosis (increased acidity) is a concern on a keto diet, as is the risk of dehydration and nausea. By combining the principles of the two diets into a keto-alkaline way of eating you can alleviate these symptoms whilst being able to experience the benefits of both.

SO, WHAT SHOULD YOU BE EATING?

A diet that's high in healthy fats, low in carbs and full of alkaline rich vegetables, and limited fruit, is the perfect way of achieving optimum hormone health.

This means that you should consume no:

- Bread and grains
- Pasta
- Sugar in any form
- Cereals
- Crisps
- Barley
- Corn
- Flour
- Couscous
- Semolina
- Cakes
- Beer
- Processed foods
- Oats
- Dried fruits
- Potatoes

But lots of:

- Alkaline vegetables such as: Artichokes, asparagus, runner beans, broccoli cabbage, carrots, celery, cauliflower, chard, aubergine, kale, leeks, lettuce, mushrooms, radish, spinach, sprouts, courgette, watercress, tomatoes and greens, avocado, lemon and limes.
- Eggs
- Nuts
- Coconut oil
- Extra-virgin olive oil
- Organic grass-fed butter
- Olives
- Seeds
- Herbs and spices
- Pickles
- Fish & shellfish

A limited amount of:

- Beetroot, parsnips and sweet potatoes
- Alkaline fruits such as: apples, apricots, bananas, berries, melon, cherries, grapes, grapefruit, mangoes, peaches, pears, pineapple and tangerines
- Free range meats
- Non-GMO soy

HOW TO BEGIN:

Insulin is one of the key hormones that affects all other hormones. If your insulin levels are out of balance, then it's likely your others will be too.

Insulin resistance is common as we approach menopause, so it becomes harder for us to cope with high levels of carbohydrates. It can lead to hot flushes as well as weight gain. The first step towards a healthy lifestyle is getting our insulin levels under control. The best way of doing this is by kick starting our systems through intermittent fasting. This essentially means swapping between periods of eating and fasting. Some people like to do this by drastically reducing calories for 2 or 3 days a week, whilst others find eating all of your daily food within a 4 to 6-hour period is best. Experiment to find the method that works best for you.

Eating this way has been shown to balance hormones, lower insulin levels, promote cellular repair, reduce belly fat, reduce inflammation, and so much more. It is just the kick-start your body needs, combined with following the keto-alkaline dietary principles, to get your body into a healthy balanced place.

In this book you will find that all of the recipes adhere to keto-alkaline principles, which will dramatically improve your hormone balance, but there are other ways that you can supplement your diet to ensure that you're in peak health. Taking a daily dose of about 400–800 IU of vitamin E has been shown by studies to reduce hot flushes, while vitamin C, magnesium glycinate (or magnesium l-threonate) and methylated B vitamins (Methyl B-Complex) have all been shown to have benefits for women who are experiencing fluctuating hormone levels.

BENEFITS OF CHANGE

By using the recipes in this book, alongside intermittent fasting for the first 10 days (the recipes that are suitable for this period will be indicated throughout) and the recommended supplements, you will be able to kick start your system into producing new hormone receptors and speed up your metabolic rate. Your hormone levels will become stabilised and you will be relieved of metabolic stall and weight gain, hot flushes, night sweats, insomnia, memory loss or brain fog, irritability, low libido, and painful sex.

By following the principles outlined above, as well as eating the delicious food that these recipes provide, you will be able to reset the efficiency of your hormones, and reverse resistance to your seven major metabolic hormones; cortisol, thyroid, testosterone, growth hormone, leptin, insulin, and oestrogen. In doing so, you will be able to counter a slowing metabolism, symptoms of aging, poor mood and sleep, and instead look forward to the next stage in your life as a woman, full of health, energy and balance.

BREAKFAST

KETO GREEN SMOOTHIE

Ingredients

- 250ml/8½floz cold water
- 250g/9oz baby spinach
- 125g/4oz coriander
- 1-inch piece fresh ginger, peeled

- ½ peeled cucumber
- ½ peeled lemon
- 1 peeled avocado

Method

1 Add all of the ingredients to a blender.

2 Blitz for approximately 30 seconds, or until smooth.

3 Top up with more water or ice if required.

4 Serve immediately.

5 Alternatively, you can store the smoothie in an air-tight container, in the fridge, for up to 3 days.

CHEF'S NOTE
This smoothie is high in alkaline vegetables and healthy fats from the avocado so it's a good breakfast to have on a fasting day.

KALE AND COCONUT SMOOTHIE

Ingredients

- 250ml/8½floz unsweetened almond milk
- 120ml/4floz full-fat coconut milk
- 200g/7oz kale, chopped
- 50g/2oz unsweetened ground coconut
- 1-inch piece peeled fresh ginger
- ¼ tsp Himalayan pink salt
- Large handful ice

Method

If you prefer a creamier smoothie, begin by blanching your kale in boiling water for 1 minute and then plunging into ice cold water, drain and squeeze out the excess water.

Pour the almond and coconut milk into base of blender.

Add the ginger, kale, ground coconut, salt and ice.

Blend until very smooth. This may take several minutes.

Serve immediately.

CHEF'S NOTE

Himalayan pink salt contains calcium, iron, potassium and magnesium and is lower in sodium than regular table salt.

TURMERIC SMOOTHIE

Ingredients

- 200ml/7floz full fat coconut milk
- 200ml/7floz unsweetened almond milk
- 1 tsp granulated sweetener
- 1 tbsp ground turmeric
- 1 tsp ground cinnamon
- 1 tsp ground ginger
- 1 tbsp coconut oil
- 1 tbsp Chia seeds
- 3-4 ice cubes

Method

1 Combine all of the ingredients, except the chia seeds, in a blender.

2 Add the ice and blend for around 30 seconds, or until smooth.

3 Pour into a glass.

4 Sprinkle chia seeds on top and enjoy straight away.

CHEF'S NOTE

Turmeric has numerous health benefits including; anti-inflammatory properties, blood sugar stabilising, helping regulate healthy periods, preventing fibroids and endometriosis, and decreasing the risk of ovarian and breast cancer!

COCONUT PANCAKES

Ingredients

- 75g/3oz full fat cream cheese
- 4 tbsp coconut flour
- 3 tbsp cream
- 2 eggs
- ½ tsp vanilla extract
- 1 tsp stevia, or another sweetener, to taste
- 1 pinch salt

Method

Mix all of the ingredients in a bowl or blender until very smooth.

Leave mixture to rest for 5 minutes to allow the coconut flour to thicken the mix and the bubbles to settle.

Fry the pancakes on a greased pan, over a medium heat, for 1-2 minutes each side until bubbles appear on the upper surface. The mix should make approximately 10 small pancakes.

CHEF'S NOTE
Coconut flour is a good alternative to wheat flour when eating a ketogenic diet. Try serving with some alkaline berries to ramp up the antioxidants.

BANANA NUT PANCAKES

Ingredients

- 2 scoops banana nut protein powder (check that your brand is unsweetened)
- 125g/4oz cream cheese
- 4 large eggs
- 1 tsp vanilla extract
- 2 tsp baking powder
- 1 tbsp stevia, or another sweetener, to taste
- Butter for cooking

Method

1 Combine all of the ingredients in a high-power blender.

2 Blend until everything is creamy and well combined. You may need to scrape down the sides with a rubber spatula and pulse again to make sure everything is completely mixed.

3 Brush a large frying pan with butter and heat over medium-low heat. Once the pan is hot, add 2 tbsp of the batter and cook until it is bubbly on top and golden brown on the bottom - this should take about 3 minutes.

4 Flip and cook the other side until it is golden brown. Repeat this process until all the batter is used.

CHEF'S NOTE

Vanilla is a great addition to a hormone balancing diet. The oil has been shown to contain antioxidant properties, boost libido, relieve PMS symptoms, prevent the growth of cancer cells, fight infection, work as an antidepressant, reduce inflammation and lower blood pressure.

GREEN OMELETTE

Ingredients

- 6 large eggs
- 1 handful kale, chopped with any thick stems removed
- 200g/7oz frozen spinach, thawed and squeezed dry
- 2 tbsp milk

- 25g/1oz mature cheddar, grated
- 25g/1oz Parmesan cheese, grated
- 125g/4oz ricotta cheese
- 25g/1oz mild feta cheese, crumbled
- 1 tbsp parsley or chives

Method

Finely chop the kale and spinach. Add the eggs, milk, cheddar and Parmesan, and mix until well combined.

Mix the feta, ricotta and chopped fresh herbs in another bowl and season with pepper. Set aside.

Heat 1 tsp of olive oil in a non-stick pan and pour in half the egg mixture. Fry on a medium heat until just set.

Add half the feta and ricotta mixture on top and gently fold the omelette over. Place a lid on the pan and cook for another minute, until the filling is warmed.

Grate some extra Parmesan on top and keep warm whilst you make the second omelette.

CHEF'S NOTE

Both kale and parsley contain properties that boost your liver's ability to metabolise oestrogen. Oestrogen increases collagen production, keeping your skin firm, taut and quick to repair.

CHOCOLATE GRANOLA

Ingredients

- 250g/9oz sliced almonds
- 250g/9oz hazelnuts, roughly chopped
- 150g/5oz unsweetened cocoa powder
- 125g/4oz pecans, rough chopped
- 125g/4oz ground flaxseed
- 125g/4oz unsweetened coconut flakes

- 60g/2½oz unsweetened cacao nibs
- ½ tsp cinnamon
- ½ tsp ground nutmeg
- 60ml/2floz sugar-free maple syrup
- 60ml/2floz coconut oil, melted
- 1 tsp pure vanilla extract

Method

1 Preheat the oven to 150C/300F/Gas Mark 2. Line a rimmed baking sheet with parchment paper.

2 Combine the almonds, hazelnuts, cocoa powder, pecans, flaxseed, coconut flakes, cacao nibs, cinnamon and nutmeg in a large mixing bowl. Mix until all ingredients are well combined.

3 In a separate bowl, combine the coconut oil, syrup, and vanilla extract. Mix until all ingredients are well incorporated.

4 Pour the coconut oil mixture over the dry ingredients and toss to coat until everything is evenly mixed and coated.

5 Spread the mixture in a single layer across the prepared baking sheet.

6 Bake for 60 minutes, tossing every 15 minutes.

7 Remove from the oven and allow to cool. The granola will continue to crisp as it cools.

CHEF'S NOTE

Chocolate may seem an odd ingredient to find in a diet book, but unsweetened cocoa contains magnesium, sulphur, calcium, iron, zinc, copper, potassium and vitamin B.

SPICED GRANOLA

Ingredients

- 250g/9oz chopped pecans
- 150g/5oz chopped walnuts
- 150g/5oz slivered almonds
- 150g/5oz unsweetened flaked coconut
- 150g/5oz ground almonds
- 60g/2½oz flax seeds
- 60g/2½oz pumpkin seeds
- 60g/2½oz sunflower seeds
- 60g/2½oz butter, melted
- 1 tsp honey
- 1 tsp cinnamon
- 1 tsp vanilla
- ½ tsp nutmeg
- ½ tsp salt
- 60ml/2floz water

Method

Preheat oven to 130C/ 250F/ Gas Mark ½.

In a large bowl, combine all of the ingredients. Mix very well.

Place a piece of parchment paper on a baking tray and grease it. Spread the granola on the tray. Place a second piece of parchment on the granola. With a rolling pin, roll the granola, to compress it into a firm and even sheet. Remove the top piece of parchment and discard.

Bake for about 60 to 90 minutes, or until golden brown. Remove from the oven and allow to fully cool before breaking into pieces.

CHEF'S NOTE

Nuts and seeds are a great addition to a ketogenic diet, as they're low in carbohydrates and high in healthy fats and protein. You can experiment with adding your favourites for a different take on this granola.

MEXICAN BREAKFAST

Ingredients

- 450g/1lb minced beef
- 4 tbsp taco seasoning (ensure it contains no added sugar)
- 175ml/6fl oz water
- 10 large eggs
- 350g/12oz cheddar cheese, grated

- 60ml/2floz double cream
- 1 large tomato, diced
- 1 medium avocado, peeled, pitted and cubed
- 60g/2½oz black olives, sliced
- 2 spring onions, sliced
- 60ml/2floz sour cream

- 60ml/2floz salsa
- 1 jalapeno, sliced
- 2 tbsp fresh coriander, tor

Method

1 Preheat the oven to 190C/375F/Gas Mark 5.

2 Brown the beef in a large pan over a medium-high heat. Drain the excess fat.

3 Add the taco seasoning and water. Reduce the heat to low and allow to simmer until the sauce has thickened and coats the meat - this should take about 5 minutes. Remove half of the seasoned beef and set aside.

4 Crack the eggs into a large mixing bowl and whisk. Add half the cheddar cheese and the cream to the eggs and whisk to combine.

5 Pour the egg mixture over top of the meat in the pan and stir to combine. Bake for 30 minutes in the oven, or until the egg bake is cooked and fluffy.

6 Top with remaining mince, cheese, tomato, avocado, olives, green onion, sour cream, and salsa.

7 Garnish with jalapeno and coriander, and serve.

CHEF'S NOTE
This dish may not be a quick midweek breakfast on the go, but is perfect for a brunch when you may be cooking for a group. Delicious and hormone balancing too.

BREAKFAST LOAF

Ingredients

- 125g/4oz peanut butter
- 125g/4oz butter, melted
- 5 eggs
- 120ml/4floz coconut or almond milk
- 1 tsp vanilla extract

- 125g/4oz ground almonds
- 2 tsp baking powder
- ½ tsp sea salt
- 125g/4oz frozen mixed berries

Method

Preheat oven to 180C/350F/Gas Mark 4. Use a silicone loaf pan, or line a loaf pan with parchment paper.

In a large mixing bowl, combine the peanut butter, melted butter and eggs. Mix until well combined.

Add the coconut milk and vanilla extract and mix well.

In a separate mixing bowl, combine the almonds, baking powder and sea salt. Mix together until well combined.

Slowly pour the wet mixture into the dry ingredients, mixing as you pour until all of the ingredients are well incorporated.

Using a rubber spatula, gently fold the mixed berries into the mixture.

7 Pour the batter into the loaf pan.

8 Bake for 45 minutes to an hour, checking on it at the 45-minute mark.

9 Remove from oven and allow to cool before slicing.

CHEF'S NOTE

This loaf is a great alternative to carb-laden, sugary muffins and will keep your insulin levels stable. Try toasting a slice and topping with butter.

CLOUD EGGS

Ingredients

- 4 large eggs
- 60g/2½oz mature cheddar cheese, grated
- 60g/2½oz sour cream
- 1 tsp garlic powder
- 2 chives, chopped
- 2 tsp salted butter

Method

1 Preheat oven to 230C/450F/Gas Mark 8.

2 Line a rimmed baking sheet with a parchment paper.

3 Separate the eggs, pouring the whites into a large mixing bowl, and the yolks into individual ramekins.

4 Using an electric hand mixer, whip the egg whites until they are fluffy and stiff peaks have started to form.

5 Using a rubber spatula, gently fold in the cheese, sour cream, garlic powder, and half of the chives.

6 Spoon the mixture into 4 separate mounds on your baking sheet. Make a well in the centre of each 'cloud' and gently pour a yolk into each one.

7 Bake for 6 minutes or until the 'clouds' are golden brown on top and the yolks are set.

8 Place a small amount of butter on top of each yolk. Top with remaining chives.

CHEF'S NOTE

Eggs are a nutrient powerhouse, containing high levels of vitamin A, folate, B vitamins, phosphorus and selenium. They are particularly good for aiding eye health as we age.

SPINACH AND FETA 'MUFFINS'

Ingredients

- 1 tbsp olive oil
- 1kg/2¼lbs baby spinach leaves, chopped
- 1 small onion, finely chopped
- 1 garlic clove, minced
- ½ green pepper, finely diced
- ½ tsp salt
- ¼ tsp black pepper

- 8 whole eggs
- 6 egg whites
- 100g/3½oz Feta cheese, crumbled
- 50g/1¾oz sundried tomatoes, finely chopped
- 1 tsp fresh thyme
- Grating of fresh nutmeg

Method

Preheat oven to 180C/350F/Gas Mark 4 and coat a 12-cup muffin pan with cooking spray, or brush lightly with olive oil.

Drizzle a large pan with olive oil, and place over medium heat. Add the onions and cook for about 4-5 minutes, stirring occasionally, until translucent and tender. Add salt, pepper, garlic and the green pepper, and continue cooking for about a minute.

Add the spinach leaves and toss gently until completely wilted. Remove from the heat and set aside.

In a large mixing bowl, add the whole eggs, egg whites, fresh thyme and nutmeg. Beat the eggs until fully incorporated and slightly frothy. Add the spinach mixture, sun dried tomatoes and Feta cheese.

5 Spoon into the prepared muffin tin. Do not fill the cups more than ¾ of the way up, to avoid spillage.

6 Cook for 22-25 minutes, until the eggs are set and top starts to colour.

7 Allow to cool on a cooling rack for at least 10 minutes before removing from the cups.

CHEF'S NOTE

These muffins are a great way to ensure you have a hormone balancing breakfast, even on busy weekdays. Make a batch when you have time and eat cold, or pop in the microwave to reheat.

STUFFED PEPPERS

Ingredients

- 4 peppers, halved and de-seeded
- 8 large eggs
- 4 rashers of bacon, diced
- 125g/4oz mushrooms, chopped
- 1 small onion, diced
- 1 garlic clove, minced
- 60g/2½oz cheddar cheese, grated

Method

1 Preheat oven to 180C/350F/Gas Mark 4.

2 Put the peppers on a baking sheet and give them a light brushing of olive oil. Sprinkle each with a little salt and pepper. Place in the oven while you prepare the rest of the ingredients.

3 In a large non-stick pan over medium heat, add the bacon and sausage. Cook until the sausage is cooked through and the bacon is crispy.

4 Add the mushrooms and onions to the pan. Continue to cook until the vegetables are tender.

5 Remove the peppers from the oven, spoon the meat mixture into them and top each pepper with cheese.

6 Using a spoon, press down in the centre of each pepper cup to create a well for the egg yolk.

7 Crack an egg over the top of each pepper.

8 Bake on the middle rack until the egg whites are cooked all the way through and the yolks have reached your desired consistency -this should take around 10 minutes.

CHEF'S NOTE

Another delicious meal that will make you the envy of guests, or simply a delicious weekend lunch for family. Peppers are antioxidant rich and great for hormone balancing.

TUNA 'MUFFINS'

Ingredients

- 2 x 175g/6oz tins tuna, drained well
- 2 eggs
- 1 celery stick, finely chopped
- 1 small onion, finely chopped
- 1 green pepper, finely chopped
- A pinch of paprika

Method

Preheat the oven to 180C/350F/Gas Mark 4.

Grease a 6-hole muffin tin.

Mix all of the ingredients together and spoon into the tin.

Bake for 30 minutes or until puffed, set and lightly browned around the edges.

Allow to cool slightly before moving from the tin.

CHEF'S NOTE

By using tuna that's canned in oil, you will increase your fat intake (perfect for a keto diet), but if you prefer your tuna canned in brine, serve with a good dollop of mayonnaise.

BAKED EGG AND HAM

Ingredients

- 1 large slice of ham
- 40g/1½oz baby spinach
- 1 medium egg

Method

1 Preheat the oven to 180C/160C Fan/Gas Mark 4.

2 Line a ramekin with the ham. Pour some boiling water into a small saucepan over a low heat. Add the spinach and cook for 2 minutes, or until wilted.

3 Remove from the heat, squeeze out any excess water and place on top of the ham.

4 Break the egg on top of the spinach.

5 Bake for 10–15 minutes, or until the egg has set, and serve.

CHEF'S NOTE
These baked eggs are a delightful start to the day and are perfect when you're fasting. They're also good as a dinner party starter.

BAKED MUSHROOMS

Ingredients

- 1 tsp olive oil
- 2 large, flat Portobello mushrooms, wiped clean, stalks finely chopped
- 1 spring onion, thinly sliced
- 1 stick celery, thinly sliced
- 2 bacon slices, roughly chopped
- 1 large handful baby spinach
- 1 beef tomato, sliced

Method

Preheat the oven to 200C/400F/Gas Mark 7.

Heat the oil in a small frying pan over a medium heat.

Add the mushroom stalks, spring onion, celery and bacon, and cook for a few minutes. Stir in the spinach and season.

Place the mushrooms cup-side up on a baking tray. Season the tomato and place on the baking tray.

Spoon the filling into the mushrooms and bake for 10–15 minutes, or until they have softened. Serve the mushrooms with the sliced tomato.

CHEF'S NOTE

These mushrooms make a hearty breakfast that's full of alkaline vegetables. Great for a fasting day, or try topping with crumbled feta on other days.

SMOKED SALMON AND SCRAMBLED EGGS

Ingredients

- 1 tsp butter
- 2 medium eggs, beaten
- 25g/1oz smoked salmon, roughly chopped
- Freshly ground black pepper

Method

1 Heat the butter in a small saucepan over a medium-low heat.

2 Season the eggs with black pepper and stir in the salmon. Pour into the saucepan.

3 Cook very gently for 3–4 minutes, stirring slowly, until the eggs are scrambled. Remove from the heat and stir for a few seconds.

4 Spoon onto a warm plate and serve.

CHEF'S NOTE

A decadent feeling breakfast that's perfect for an alkaline-keto diet and good for fast days too. Experiment by adding in some wilted spinach or cream cheese.

BREAKFAST TRAY BAKE

Ingredients

- 8 eggs
- 2 red peppers, de-seeded and finely sliced
- 75g/3oz chestnut mushrooms, halved and thinly sliced
- 40g/1½oz spinach, roughly chopped
- 50g/2oz mature cheddar cheese, grated
- ½ tsp sea salt
- Freshly ground black pepper

Method

Preheat the oven to 180C/350F/Gas Mark 4.

Lightly grease a 35cm/14 in x 25cm/10in 2cm/¾in deep roasting tin and line with baking paper.

Crack the eggs into a large bowl, add the salt and pepper, and whisk well.

Pour the eggs into the roasting tin, making sure they spread into the corners. Scatter the peppers, mushrooms and spinach over the eggs and top with the cheddar.

Place in the oven to bake for 10–12 minutes, or until just set and lightly golden around the edges.

Remove the eggs from the oven and leave to rest for 2 minutes, then slide out onto a board and cut into pieces.

CHEF'S NOTE

This dish is perfect, no matter whether you have it fresh from the oven for breakfast, a cold slice for lunch, or even warm with a side salad for dinner.

BREAKFAST FRITTATA

Ingredients

- 2 rashers back bacon
- 125g/4oz mushrooms, thinly sliced
- 75g/3oz spinach
- 100g/3½oz cherry tomatoes, halved
- 4 eggs, beaten

Method

1 Preheat the grill to medium-high. Grill the bacon until it is browned on both sides. Remove and set aside.

2 Spray a small non-stick frying pan with oil and place on a medium-high heat. Fry the mushrooms for 5 minutes, stirring frequently, until they are browned and softened. Set aside.

3 Rinse the spinach under cold water and drain it in a sieve. Add it to the frying pan and cook for 1-2 minutes, stirring all the time. When the spinach is wilted transfer back to the sieve and press with the back of a spoon to squeeze any remaining water from the leaves. Set aside.

4 Wipe the frying pan clean, spray with oil and fry the tomatoes for about 5 minutes.

5 Beat the eggs in a fairly large bowl. Chop the cooked bacon and the spinach. Add to the eggs, along with the cooked mushrooms, and season with salt and freshly ground black pepper.

6 When the tomatoes are cooked, spoon them into the eggs with the other vegetables. Give the egg mixture a brief stir, then pour it back into the frying pan and place it over the heat. Cook gently on a medium heat for 10 minutes, until the egg looks set around the edges (it may be a little runny on the top).

7 Place the pan under the grill for 2 minutes to finish cooking the frittata on top. Turn it out onto a plate and let it cool slightly before cutting into wedges to serve..

CAJUN SCRAMBLED EGGS

Ingredients

- 4 large eggs
- 75ml/2½floz single cream
- ½ red onion, finely chopped
- 1 large green pepper, seeds removed and finely chopped

- 40g/1½ oz kale, shredded
- 1½ tsp Cajun spice mix (ensure there is no added sugar)
- 50g/2oz spinach leaves

Method

Beat together the eggs and cream with salt and pepper.

Add a few sprays of oil to a large non-stick frying pan and warm over a medium heat. Add the onion and green pepper, and cook for 3–4 minutes, or until slightly softened.

Add the kale with a dash of water and cook for 2 minutes. Sprinkle over the Cajun spice mix, a pinch of salt and the spinach. Cook, stirring frequently, for 1 minute, or until the spinach has wilted.

Add another few sprays of oil to the pan. Pour in the egg mixture and let it set for a few seconds, then gently stir until scrambled and just cooked.

Spoon onto warmed plates and serve.

CHEF'S NOTE

Spinach is one of the best ingredients for balancing your thyroid hormones. It's rich in iron and B vitamins, which can help give you a boost if you're tired. Ideal for a fast day.

TURKISH EGGS

Ingredients

- 200g/7oz Greek yoghurt
- 1 garlic clove, crushed
- 1 tsp sea salt flakes
- 2 tbsp butter

- 1 tbsp extra virgin olive oil
- 1 tsp chilli flakes
- 2 large free-range eggs, fridge cold

Method

1 Fill a saucepan with around 4cm/1½in of water and bring to the boil. Place the yoghurt into a heatproof bowl large enough to sit over the pan, and stir in the garlic and salt. Place the bowl over the pan, making sure the base doesn't touch the water. Stir until it reaches body temperature and has the consistency of lightly whipped double cream. Turn off the heat, leaving the bowl over the pan.

2 Melt the butter gently in a separate saucepan, until it is just beginning to turn brown. Turn the heat off, then stir in the oil, followed by the chilli flakes, and set aside.

3 Fill a wide, lidded saucepan with 4cm/1½in of water and place over a medium heat. When it is just starting to simmer, gently slide in the eggs,

one on each side of the pan. Turn the heat down low and poach the eggs for 3–4 minutes, until the whites are set, but the yolks are still runny. Using slotted spoon, gently transfer the eggs to a plate lined with kitchen roll.

4 Divide the warm, creamy yoghurt between two shallow bowls, top each with a poached egg and the melted butter.

CHEF'S NOTE

Eating enough protein is important step in ensuring the hormone that controls your appetite (ghrelin) is kept under control. Eggs are packed full of protein, keeping you feeling full for longer.

LUNCH & LIGHT MEALS

CREAMY COURGETTI

Ingredients

- 1 ripe avocado
- 1 garlic clove
- Large bunch fresh basil leaves
- 1 tbsp lemon juice
- 2 tbsp extra virgin olive oil
- 2-3 courgettes, spiralized or cut into ¼ inch wide strips

Method

1 First, make the sauce by blending the avocado, garlic, basil leaves and lemon juice in a food processor until smooth, then mix in extra virgin olive oil. Add water, 1 tbsp at a time, until the sauce reaches a fluid yet thick consistency. Season with salt and pepper to taste.

2 Sauté the courgette with a splash of olive oil over medium/high heat, until slightly soft and bright green - usually around 3 to 5 minutes. Drain the excess water.

3 Toss the courgette with the sauce, then top with parmesan cheese.

CHEF'S NOTE
Adapting to cutting carbs from your diet can seem difficult at first, but there are easy substitutes that can be made, such as substituting pasta for courgettes in this creamy, zesty dish.

MEXICAN SOUP

Ingredients

- 675g/1½lbs boneless skinless chicken breasts
- 1 tbsp olive oil
- 6 spring onions, finely sliced
- 2 jalapeños, finely chopped
- 2 garlic cloves, minced
- 2lt/3pts chicken stock
- 2 large tomatoes, seeded and diced
- ½ tsp ground cumin
- 1 large handful chopped coriander
- 3 tbsp fresh lime juice
- 3 medium avocados, peeled and diced

Method

In a large saucepan, heat 1 tbsp olive oil over medium heat. Once hot, add the onions and jalapeños and sauté for around 2 minutes, or until tender, adding garlic during last 30 seconds.

Add the chicken stock, tomatoes and cumin, then season with salt and pepper before adding the chicken breasts.

Bring the mixture to a boil over medium-high heat, then reduce the heat to medium, cover with a lid and allow to cook, stirring occasionally, until the chicken has cooked through – usually around 10 - 15 minutes.

Reduce the heat to low, remove the chicken from pan and allow to rest on a cutting board for 5 minutes.

5 Shred the chicken and return it to the soup. Stir in the coriander and lime juice.

6 Add the diced avocado to the soup just before serving.

CHEF'S NOTE
This fiery soup is packed with protein and good fats, yet tastes surprisingly light. Good for a fast day, but you can top with sour cream and grated cheese on other days, if desired.

KALE SOUP WITH TURKEY MEATBALLS

Ingredients

For the meatballs:
- **450g/1lb turkey mince**
- **1 egg, beaten**
- **2 garlic cloves, crushed**
- **2 tbsp fresh herbs (parsley, basil, dill, or coriander)**

- **2 tbsp butter, ghee, or coconut oil**

For the soup:
- **2 tbsp butter, ghee, or coconut oil**
- **1 onion, diced**
- **4 large carrots, chopped**
- **2 garlic cloves, minced**

- **2 bay leaves**
- **2lt/3pts chicken stock**
- **1 bunch kale, de-stemmed and chopped**

Method

1 First, make the meatballs by combining the mince, egg, garlic, salt, and herbs, then mix until well. Roll into small balls. This should make 24-26 meatballs.

2 Heat 2 tbsp of the fat of your choice in a large frying pan on a medium-high heat. Cook the meatballs for 3-4 minutes, until all sides are brown. You may need to do this in batches. Set aside.

3 Heat 2 tbsp of the fat of your choice in large soup pot. Add the onions, carrots and garlic, and cook until the onions are translucent – usually about 5 minutes.

4 Add the bay leaves, stock and meatballs. Bring to a boil, turn down the heat and simmer for 5 minutes.

5 Add the kale and cook for a further 5-7 minutes, until the meatballs are cooked through.

6 Serve immediately.

CHEF'S NOTE

Turkey is an underused meat, but a wonderful source of protein. This dish also contains hormone-balancing healthy fats, antioxidant rich vegetables and healing herbs and spices.

ASIAN SALAD

Ingredients

For the Salad:
- 4 eggs
- 150g/5oz cherry tomatoes
- 500g/1lb 2oz Chinese greens
- 1 medium cauliflower, diced
- 250g/9oz beansprouts
- 175g/6oz silken tofu, diced

- 1 tbsp sesame oil
- ½ cucumber, sliced

For the dressing:
- 125g/4oz crunchy peanut butter
- 2 limes, juice only
- 1 garlic clove

- 1 fresh red chilli, deseeded
- 2 tsp Asian fish sauce
- 1 tbsp soy sauce
- To Garnish:
- Crushed peanuts
- Coriander

Method

Begin by frying the tofu in the sesame oil on a medium heat for 15 minutes. Meanwhile halve the tomatoes and chop the chinese greens.

Whilst the tofu is frying, carefully lower the eggs into boiling water and boil for 6 minutes, or until nearly hard boiled. Remove from the hot water and place in bowl of cold water. Once cooled, peel and cut each egg in half.

Boil or steam the cauliflower for 3-4 minutes then remove from the water and allow to cool whilst preparing the other ingredients.

To prepare the sauce, place all the ingredients in a blender and blitz until you have a well combined, fairly smooth sauce. Season with extra salt and lime juice to taste

5 Add the tofu and cauliflower to the rest of the salad ingredients (except the eggs), pour over the sauce and mix everything thoroughly.

6 Top with the halved eggs, coriander and crushed peanuts.

CHEF'S NOTE
This dish transports well, making it a good choice if you wish to prepare lunch in advance for work or a picnic. Try substituting the tofu for chicken, pork or prawns for a non-veggie version.

MEXICAN SALAD

Ingredients

- 450g/1lb minced beef
- 4 tbsp taco seasoning (ensure no added sugar)
- 400g/14oz tinned chopped tomatoes with chilli
- 200g/7oz carrots, shredded
- 150g/5oz white cabbage, shredded
- 125g/4oz black olives, sliced
- 1 large avocado, peeled, pitted and sliced
- 2 spring onions, sliced
- Fresh coriander or flat-leaf parsley (optional)
- Sliced jalapeños (optional)
- Sour cream (optional)

Method

1 Heat a large frying pan over a medium heat. Put the minced beef and 2 tbsp of the seasoning blend in the pan and cook for about 15 minutes, or until the meat is browned and cooked through.

2 Add the chopped tomatoes, shredded carrots and cabbage, and the remaining 2 tbsp of the seasoning blend. Cook for around 5-7 minutes, until the cabbage is tender.

3 Stir in the olives and cook until thoroughly heated. Taste and add salt, if needed.

4 Top each serving with the avocado slices and spring onions, as well as the coriander, jalapeños and sour cream, if using.

CHEF'S NOTE

Beef is a great food to eat as part of an alkaline-keto diet, but it's important to look at where it comes from. Grass-fed beef can contain between 2 and 5 times more Omega-3 than grain-fed beef.

SERVES 1

BEETROOT AND FETA SALAD

Ingredients

- 50g/2oz green beans
- 100g/3½oz beetroot, cooked
- 1 large handful baby spinach
- 40g/1½ oz feta cheese, crumbled

Method

Simmer the green beans in water over a medium heat for 4–5 minutes.

Drain and rinse under cold running water until cool.

Toss the beans with the beetroot and spinach in a small bowl.

Top with the cheese and serve.

CHEF'S NOTE

This is a quick and easy salad to throw together for lunch, or as an accompaniment to roast or grilled meats. It would go particularly well with left over roast lamb.

SPICED CHICKEN SALAD

Ingredients

- 100g/3½oz pre-prepared, cooked chicken tikka, sliced (ensure no added sugar)
- 50g/2oz salad leaves
- 50g/2oz cucumber, thinly sliced
- 2 spring onions, thinly sliced
- 1 handful fresh coriander, roughly chopped (optional)
- 1 tbsp tzatziki (ensure no added sugar)

Method

1 Combine the chicken, cucumber, spring onions and coriander in a bowl.

2 Spread the salad over a plate and top with the other ingredients.

3 Drizzle the tzatziki on top.

4 Serve immediately, or keep in the fridge for a few hours.

CHEF'S NOTE

This salad is a great way of using up leftovers that you may have hanging about. Spiced but not hot, this dish is quick enough to make in the morning before work.

PRAWN COUSCOUS SALAD

Ingredients

- 100g/3½oz cauliflower florets
- 1 tsp olive oil
- 100g/3½oz prawns, peeled and cooked
- 1 large tomato, roughly chopped
- ¼ onion medium, finely chopped

- ½ tsp olive oil
- Pinch of dried red chilli flakes
- 1 small bunch fresh coriander, roughly chopped (optional)

Method

Preheat the oven to 200C/400F Fan/Gas 6.

To make the cauliflower 'couscous' pulse the cauliflower in a food processor for 30 seconds, or until finely chopped. Mix in the oil and season to taste. Spread the couscous onto a baking tray and bake for 15 minutes.

Whilst the cauliflower is cooking, mix all of the remaining ingredients together.

Serve the prawn mix with the 'couscous', either hot or cool.

CHEF'S NOTE

Replacing carbohydrates which destabilise blood sugars is key to healthy weight loss. Cauliflower is an ideal substitute for couscous, rice or other grains.

GREEK SALAD

Ingredients

- ½ small red onion, thinly sliced
- 2 large ripe tomatoes, roughly chopped
- ½ cucumber, deseeded and roughly chopped
- 100g/3½oz reduced fat feta cheese, drained and cut into cubes
- 50g/2oz black olives, pitted and drained
- 1 small handful fresh mint leaves
- ½ tsp dried oregano
- 2 tsp extra virgin olive oil
- 2 tsp fresh lemon juice

Method

1 Put the onion, tomatoes and cucumber in a bowl and season to taste.

2 Scatter over the feta, olives, mint leaves and oregano, then toss lightly.

3 Drizzle over the oil and lemon juice to serve.

CHEF'S NOTE

A tasty light lunch or main meal accompaniment. Olives and olive oil both contain high levels of hormone-balancing, healthy fats.

WALDORF SALAD

Ingredients

- 2 crunchy red apples, cored and sliced
- ½ lemon, juice only
- 150g/5oz red and green seedless grapes, halved
- 2 celery sticks, thinly sliced
- 4 spring onions, thinly sliced

- 1 little gem lettuce, leaves separated and roughly torn
- 350g/12oz chicken breasts, cooked and roughly torn
- 2 tbsp toasted walnuts, chopped

For the dressing:
- 200g/7oz natural yoghurt
- 1 garlic clove, crushed
- 1 tbsp cider vinegar
- 1 level tbsp wholegrain mustard
- 2–3 tbsp chopped fresh dill

Method

Place the apples in a wide salad bowl and toss with the lemon juice. Add the grapes, celery, spring onion, lettuce and chicken, and toss again.

To make the dressing, whisk the yoghurt, garlic, vinegar, mustard and dill together, and season. Spoon the dressing over the salad and toss well.

Scatter with the walnuts and garnish with the dill to serve.

CHEF'S NOTE
This classic New York salad is rich and creamy. Walnuts are full of vitamins and minerals, as well as healthy fats to keep your home levels balanced.

CHICKEN CAESAR SALAD

Ingredients

For the Salad:
- 4 slices prosciutto
- 2 chicken breasts, bone and skin removed
- 2 cos lettuces

For the dressing:
- 2 garlic cloves

- 75ml/2½fl oz white wine
- 2 egg yolks
- 1 anchovy fillet
- 75g/3oz parmesan cheese, grated
- 150ml/5floz extra virgin olive oil
- 2 tsp Dijon mustard

Method

1 Preheat your grill to a high heat.

2 Put the prosciutto onto a baking sheet and place under the grill for 3-4 mins, or until crisp. Remove and place on a plate lined with kitchen paper to drain.

3 Butterfly the chicken breasts to open up and form one large flat piece. Season, to taste, with salt and black pepper, then brush with olive oil.

4 Heat a griddle pan until hot, then cook the chicken breasts for a few minutes on each side, or until cooked through.

5 Separate the leaves from the lettuce and cut into chunky pieces.

6 For the dressing, bring the garlic and wine to a boil in a medium saucepan, and simmer for about 5 mins, until the garlic has softened. Leave to cool.

7 Combine the wine and garlic with the egg yolks, anchovy and cheese in a mixing bowl. Blend with a hand blender or food processor until smooth. Drizzle in the oil in a thin steady stream, taking care not to add it too quickly, otherwise it could split and curdle. Stir in the mustard and add seasoning to taste.

8 Add the crispy prosciutto and lettuce to the dressing and toss to combine.

9 To serve, place the salad on plate, top with the chicken, then pour over the dressing .

BEEF CARPACCIO WITH ARTICHOKE SALAD

Ingredients

For the carpaccio:
- 300g/11oz beef fillet, trimmed
- 1 tbsp olive oil
- 2 tsp fresh oregano, chopped
- 1-2tbsp extra virgin olive oil

For the artichoke salad:
- 2 lemons, juice only

- 4-6 baby violet artichokes, trimmed
- 250g/9oz Jerusalem artichokes, peeled
- 2 tsp Dijon mustard
- 2 tbsp white wine vinegar
- 6 tbsp extra virgin olive oil

- 2 tbsp olive oil
- 4 tbsp flatleaf parsley, roughly chopped
- 3 tbsp pine nuts, toasted

Method

For the beef carpaccio, season the beef fillet with salt and freshly ground black pepper. Heat a frying pan until smoking hot, add the olive oil and sear the beef on all sides for 2-3 minutes, or until golden-brown on the outside..

Remove the beef from the pan and roll in the chopped oregano to coat. Cover in cling film and roll into a barrel shape, twisting tightly at both ends to seal, then place into the freezer for one hour, or until firm.

For the artichoke salad, thinly slice the baby violet artichokes and Jerusalem artichokes, then place them into a bowl of water with half of the lemon juice, to prevent browning.

Whisk together the mustard, vinegar and remaining lemon juice in a small bowl, then add in the extra virgin olive oil until well combined.

5 Drain the artichokes, then mix in the parsley and pine nuts. Drizzle over the dressing and mix well to coat.

6 To serve, slice the beef as thinly as possible, then arrange around the edges of a serving plate. Pile the artichoke salad into the centre of the plate.

7 Drizzle the beef with a little extra virgin olive oil and season, to taste, with salt and freshly ground black pepper.

SALMON CEVICHE

Ingredients

- 250g/9oz organic salmon fillet, skinned
- 2 tbsp rock salt
- 1 tbsp red chillies, finely diced
- 75ml/2½fl oz pink grapefruit juice
- 1 tbsp lime zest

- 150ml/5floz lime juice (about 5 limes)
- Large handful of coriander leaves, finely chopped
- 1 fennel bulb, finely sliced
- 125g/4oz baby salad leaves

Method

1 For the ceviche, lightly sprinkle the salmon fillet with rock salt. Transfer to the fridge and leave for 20 minutes.

2 Remove the salmon from the fridge, carefully wash off all the salt and pat dry.

3 In a small bowl, mix the chillies, grapefruit juice, lime zest and juice together. Add the coriander at the last minute and toss to combine.

4 Slice the salmon at an angle - each piece needs to be about 2-3mm thick.

5 Lay four slices evenly in a straight line on each serving plate.

6 Spoon all but two tablespoons of the ceviche dressing over the salmon. Set aside for about 30 minutes while it 'cooks' in the line juice.

7 For the salad, soak the sliced fennel in iced water for 2-3 minutes, before removing and draining. Mix with the salad leaves and the reserved two tablespoons of ceviche dressing.

8 Place the fennel salad on top of the salmon and serve.

CHEF'S NOTE

Salmon is an excellent source of Vitamin D, a fat-soluble vitamin that helps us make our sex hormones and boosts testosterone levels. It's also important for bone health and immunity.

GAZPACHO

Ingredients

- 1kg/2¼ lb ripe plum tomatoes, washed and halved
- 3 tbsp olive oil
- 3 garlic cloves, unpeeled and 1 garlic clove, peeled

- 1 large handful basil leaves
- 1 tbsp pine nuts
- 2 tbsp olive oil

Method

Preheat the oven to 180C/350F/Gas Mark 4

Place the tomatoes, cut side up, in a baking tray and add the unpeeled garlic cloves. Season well with salt and pepper and drizzle over the olive oil. Roast for about 45 minutes, or until the tomatoes are lightly browned and beginning to ooze juice. Remove from the oven and leave to cool for a few moments.

Pick out the roasted garlic cloves and squeeze the soft flesh out of the skin onto a plate. Place a sieve over a bowl and rub the tomatoes through it to extract the juice and flesh. Rub the roasted garlic pulp through the sieve as well, along with any oily juices from the pan.

Place the bowl in the fridge and chill for at least 4 hours.

5 Chop together the basil, garlic and pine nuts until you have a fine-grained pulp. Stir into the olive oil.

6 Serve the soup in chilled bowls, drizzled with a generous tablespoon of the pesto.

CHEF'S NOTE

This is a fresh soup that's perfect for a warm summer's day. Roasting the tomatoes adds a freshness, while the pesto is zingy and full of thyroid-balancing basil.

CREAMY CHOWDER

Ingredients

- 25g/1oz butter
- 1 tbsp sunflower oil
- 1 medium onion, chopped
- 20g/¾oz ground almonds
- 400ml/14floz semi-skimmed milk
- 400ml/14floz just-boiled water
- 100g/3½oz frozen sweetcorn
- 1 medium leek, trimmed and finely sliced
- 4 large smoked haddock fillets

Method

1 Heat the butter and oil in a large, non-stick frying pan over a medium heat. Add the onion and fry for 3 minutes, until completely softened. Sprinkle over the ground almonds and stir well.

2 In a measuring jug, mix the milk and water. Gradually add 700ml/1¼ pints of the liquid to the onions, stirring after each addition. Bring the mixture to the boil, reduce the heat and simmer, stirring regularly, for 10-12 minutes before adding the sweetcorn and leeks.

3 Place the smoked haddock fillets on top of the chowder and continue to simmer for 10-15 minutes, or until the fish is cooked and flakes eas

4 Carefully remove the cooked fish from the chowder using a slotted spoon and set aside on a warm place. Stir the remaining milk and water into the pan and return to a simmer until warmed through.

5 To serve, spoon the chowder into warm bowls, seasoning again with salt and pepper. Top each serving with one of the haddock fillets.

CHEF'S NOTE
Ground almonds are a good substitute for flour and contain nutritious fat that will help to balance blood sugar levels, aid the nervous system and combat inflammation.

TOM YUM SOUP

Ingredients

- 75g/3oz raw king prawns
- 300ml/10½floz vegetable stock
- 1 spring onion, chopped
- 1 red chilli, finely sliced

- 4 button mushrooms, thinly sliced
- ½ lime, juice only
- 1 tbsp fish sauce
- Small bunch coriander

Method

Place the stock in a saucepan and bring to the boil.

Add the chilli, mushrooms, lime juice, fish sauce and the white parts of the spring onion. Bring back to the boil, then reduce the heat and simmer for 1 minute.

Add the prawns to the stock. Simmer for another 2 minutes, or until the prawns turn pink and are cooked all the way through.

Pour the soup into a deep bowl, then stir in the green parts of the spring onion and the coriander leaves.

CHEF'S NOTE

Prawns are rich in vitamin E, which is essential to the production of sex hormones and increases blood flow and oxygen to the genital area.

GRILLED COURGETTE AND MINT FRITTATA

Ingredients

- 4 tsp olive oil
- 1 red onion, thinly sliced
- 375g/13oz courgettes, diced

- 6 eggs
- 2 tbsp chopped mint

Method

1 Heat the oil in a large, non-stick frying pan. Add the onion and courgettes, and fry over gentle heat for 5 minutes, or until lightly browned and just cooked.

2 Preheat the grill to a hot setting.

3 Beat together the eggs, 2 tablespoons of water and the chopped mint. Season with salt and freshly ground black pepper.

4 Add the egg mixture to the frying pan. Cook, without stirring, for 4-5 minutes, or until the frittata is almost set and the underside is golden brown.

5 Transfer the pan to a hot grill and cook for 3-4 minutes, or until the top is golden and the frittata cooked through.

6 Cut into wedges and serve.

CHEF'S NOTE

Eggs are full of omega 3 fatty acids, the anti-inflammatory fats that support the brain. This is wonderful to eat on fast days, perhaps served with a simple salad.

OVEN BAKED SALMON FRITTATA

Ingredients

- 6 eggs
- 2 tbsp milk
- 60g/2½oz smoked salmon trimmings
- 1 tbsp oil
- 85g/3¼oz broccoli florets, thinly sliced
- 100g/3½oz frozen peas

Method

Preheat the oven to 180C/375F/Gas Mark 4

Crack the eggs into a bowl, add the milk and a pinch of salt and pepper, then whisk. Stir in the smoked salmon.

Heat half the oil in a large ovenproof frying pan over a medium-high heat. Fry the broccoli for 3 minutes, then add the peas and fry for a further minute.

Add the remaining oil, shake the pan to evenly distribute the greens, then turn the heat up to high. Pour in the egg mixture and cook for 1 minute.

Reduce the heat to medium and fry for 2-3 minutes, or until the base is cooked and golden.

6 Bake the frittata for 10-12 minutes, or until the top is bubbled up and the frittata is fairly firm. Leave to cool.

7 Slide the frittata onto a plate, cut it into slices and serve.

CHEF'S NOTE

Broccoli is a member of the cruciferous family of vegetables, which also includes cauliflower, kale, cabbage and Brussel sprouts. It's full of nutrients which can help prevent oestrogen related cancers.

SALT AND PEPPER CHICKEN

Ingredients

- 1 tbsp fine salt
- 1 tbsp Chinese five-spice powder
- 1 tbsp ground black pepper, plus an extra tsp
- 200ml/7floz vegetable oil, plus an extra 1 tbsp

- 4 boneless, skinless, chicken thighs, cut into bite-sized strips
- 3 spring onions, thinly sliced
- 1 red finger chilli, thinly sliced
- 2 garlic cloves, crushed

Method

1 In a large bowl, mix the salt, five spice and the tablespoon of pepper together, then set aside.

2 In a wok or large pan, heat the oil to 180C/350F (use a cooking thermometer).

3 Toss the chicken in the spice mixture, working in batches. Carefully add it to the oil and cook for 2–3 minutes on each side, until golden brown and cooked though. Drain on kitchen paper.

4 Heat the remaining tablespoon of oil in a clean pan over a medium heat. Add the spring onions, chilli, garlic and remaining teaspoon of pepper with a pinch of salt. Fry for 1–2 minutes, then add the cooked chicken.

5 Toss and cook for a further 2–3 minutes, until the chicken is coated in the onions, garlic and chilli. Serve straight away.

CHEF'S NOTE

This Chinese style dish lacks the sugar and cornflour that are usually found in takeaway dishes. This is perfect for a light meal, or can be bulked out with egg-fried cauliflower rice.

SALMON NIÇOISE

Ingredients

- 900g/2lb salmon fillet
- 1 tbsp cracked black peppercorns
- 2 tbsp light olive oil
- 1 yellow pepper
- ½ tbsp vegetable oil
- 2 plum tomatoes
- 175g/6oz green beans, cooked

- 20 olives
- 2 tbsp virgin olive oil
- 2 tbsp chopped parsley
- For the dressing:
- ½ tsp salt
- 1½ tbsp Dijon mustard
- 4 tsp lemon juice

- 1 garlic clove, crushed
- 5 drops Tabasco sauce
- 4 anchovy filets
- 120ml/4floz olive oil
- 1 egg, yolk only

Method

Cut the salmon into 4 equal steaks. Sprinkle each with salt and black pepper. Coat lightly in oil and refrigerate until ready to cook.

Rub the yellow pepper with a little vegetable oil, then grill or roast until the skin is well blistered. Allow to cool, and then peel off the charred skin, remove the seeds, slice into 8 pieces and place in a bowl. Cut the tomatoes into 6 wedges each.

Combine all of the vegetables, season lightly with salt and pepper, and toss with the olive oil and parsley. Leave to come to room temperature.

To make the dressing, combine all the dressing ingredients in a blender, and pulse until smooth and emulsified.

To cook the salmon, heat a large grill pan over high heat until almost smoking. Add the salmon, and sear for 1-3 minutes on each side.

6 To serve, divide the vegetables among the plates and place a salmon steak in the centre of each. Surround with a generous drizzle of the dressing and serve immediately.

CHEF'S NOTE

Salmon is an excellent source of Vitamin D, a fat-soluble vitamin that helps us make our sex hormones and boosts testosterone levels.

STEAK TARTARE

Ingredients

- 100g/3½oz beef fillet, finely chopped
- 2 gherkins, finely chopped
- 1 tsp capers, drained, rinsed and finely chopped
- 1 shallot, finely chopped
- ½ tsp Dijon mustard
- A few drops Tabasco sauce
- ½ tsp Worcestershire sauce
- 1 egg, yolk only

Method

1 Place the chopped beef, gherkins, capers and shallot into a bowl and mix well.

2 Add the mustard, Tabasco sauce, Worcestershire sauce, salt and freshly ground black pepper, then mix well.

3 To serve, spoon the steak tartare mixture onto a plate. Make a small dent in the top of the tartare and top with a fresh egg yolk. Eat immediately.

CHEF'S NOTE

This simple yet decadent dish is all about the quality of the ingredients, so buy the best you can. Ensure your beef is organic and grass-fed, and your eggs are free range organic.

DINNER

MUSHROOM TACOS

Ingredients

- 450g/1lb portobello mushrooms
- 60g/2½oz spicy harissa
- 3 tbsp olive oil

- 1 tsp ground cumin
- 1 tsp onion powder
- 6 whole leaves from a round lettuce

Method

1 Remove the stems from the mushrooms.

2 Mix the harissa, 1½ tbsp olive oil, cumin, and onion powder in a bowl. Brush each mushroom with the harissa mixture, making sure to cover the edges as well. Let them marinade for 15 minutes.

3 Once the mushrooms have marinated, heat the rest of olive oil in a frying pan over a medium-high heat. Place the portobello mushrooms in the pan and cook for 3 minutes. Flip over and cook for a few minutes until tender. Each side should be browned.

4 Turn off the heat and let the mushrooms rest for a few minutes before slicing.

5 Take a lettuce leaf and fill it with a few mushroom slices to serve.

CHEF'S NOTE
Perfect for fast days, or vegan diners, feel free to add chilli sauce, cheese, sour cream or avocado to taste.

VEGAN CHILLI

Ingredients

- 2 tbsp extra virgin olive oil
- 5 stalks celery, finely diced
- 2 cloves garlic, minced
- 1½ tsp ground cinnamon
- 2 tsp chili powder
- 4 tsp ground cumin
- 1½ tsp smoked paprika

- 2 green peppers, finely diced
- 2 courgettes, diced
- 225g/8oz button mushrooms
- 1½ tbsp tomato paste
- 1 425g/15oz tin chopped tomatoes
- 750ml/1¼pt water

- 120ml/4floz coconut milk
- 600g/1lb 5oz soy meat, crumbled
- 250g/9oz raw walnuts, minced
- 1tbsp unsweetened cocoa powder

Method

Heat the oil in a large pot over medium heat. Add the celery and cook for 4 minutes.

Add in the garlic, cinnamon, cumin and paprika and stir for another 2 minutes, until fragrant.

Add the peppers, courgettes and mushrooms, and cook for 5 minutes.

Add the tomato paste, tomatoes, water, coconut milk, soy meat, walnuts and cocoa powder.

Reduce the heat to medium-low and simmer for about 20-25 minutes, until the sauce is thick, and the vegetables are soft.

Season with salt and pepper, to taste.

CHEF'S NOTE

It can appear difficult to cater for vegans when following a keto diet, but this chilli is so tasty you won't miss the meat!

CHICKEN STIR FRY

Ingredients

- 2 tbsp coconut oil
- 4 chicken thigh fillets, cubed
- 125g/4oz peanuts
- 1 green pepper, cut into chunks
- ½ medium white onion, cut into large chunks
- 1 medium broccoli, chopped into florets

- 2 garlic cloves, crushed
- 1-inch piece of fresh ginger, grated
- 1 tbsp rice wine vinegar
- 1 tbsp toasted sesame oil
- 1 tbsp sriracha (or other hot sauce)
- 1 tbsp sesame seeds
- 1 tbsp spring onion, chopped

Method

1 Heat oil in a hot pan, add the chicken thighs and sauté for 5-6 minutes, or until browned.

2 Add the onion, pepper and broccoli and sauté for 2-3 minutes, stirring regularly.

3 Add the garlic, peanuts, ginger and remaining liquid ingredients and sauté for a further 2-3 minutes, or until the chicken is cooked through.

4 Serve immediately, sprinkled with the chopped spring onions and sesame seeds.

CHEF'S NOTE

This stir fry is a delicious and quick mid-week meal. Broccoli is high in fibre, which helps eliminate excess oestrogen.

GARLIC CHICKEN

Ingredients

- 2 tbsp olive oil
- 4 chicken thighs, skin on
- 75g/3oz butter
- 225g/8oz green beans
- 4 garlic cloves, minced
- 1 tsp dried oregano

- 1 tsp dried rosemary
- 1 tsp dried thyme
- 1 tbsp Dijon/wholegrain mustard
- 1 lemon, juice only
- ½ lemon, peel only
- Small bunch parsley

Method

Pat the chicken dry with a paper towel, especially the skin side, then sprinkle the skin with a little salt.

Heat a frying pan on a medium heat. Once it's hot, add a tablespoon of olive oil and half the butter. Once the butter is bubbling, lay the chicken skin side down. Press each one down gently to ensure good contact with the pan and cook for 6-8 minutes, or until the skin has begun to crisp up.

In the meantime, prepare your sauce; In a bowl, combine the mustard, 1 tbsp of olive oil, dried herbs, crushed garlic, lemon zest juice, along with a little salt and pepper.

4 Flip the chicken over and cook for a further 6-10 minutes, or until it is cooked through. Remove from the pan.

5 Add the green beans into the pan and cook for 2 minutes. Then, add in the garlic and herb mixture, along with the remaining butter and cook for another 2-3 minutes, until the green beans begin to soften.

6 Add the chicken and most of the chopped parsley just before serving, keeping a little to one side to garnish on top, then serve whilst hot and crispy.

CASHEW CHICKEN

Ingredients

- 3 boneless chicken thighs
- 2 tbsp coconut oil
- 125g/4oz raw cashews
- 1 green pepper, de-seeded
- ½ tsp ground ginger
- 1 tbsp rice wine vinegar

- ½ tsp chilli flakes
- 1 tbsp garlic, minced
- 1 tbsp sesame oil
- 1 tbsp sesame seeds
- 1 tbsp spring onions
- 1 medium white onion

Method

1 Place a frying pan over low heat and toast the cashews for a few minutes, or until they start to lightly brown and become fragrant. Remove and set aside.

2 Dice the chicken thighs into 1 inch chunks. Cut the onion and pepper into equally large chunks.

3 Increase the heat to high and add the coconut oil to pan.

4 Once the oil is up to temperature, add in the chicken thighs and allow them to cook through for about 5-10 minutes.

5 Once the chicken is fully cooked, add in the pepper, onion, garlic, chilli, ginger and season well. Allow to cook on high for 2-3 minutes.

6 Add the rice wine vinegar and cashews. Cook on high and allow the liquid to reduce down until it is a sticky consistency.

7 Serve in a bowl, topped with sesame seeds and drizzled with sesame oil.

CHEF'S NOTE
Peppers are full of Vitamin C, an antioxidant essential to the function of the adrenal glands. Green peppers have less sugar than red, so are good for keto dieters.

FISH CURRY

Ingredients

- 2 tsp olive oil
- 3 cloves garlic, finely chopped
- 3cm ginger, finely chopped
- 1 green chilli, de-seeded
- 2 tomatoes
- 1 onion, finely chopped

- 1 tbsp coconut oil, melted
- 1 tbsp garam masala
- 1 tbsp ground cumin
- 1 tbsp turmeric
- 450ml/15½floz full fat coconut milk

- ½ tsp salt
- 1 lime, juice only
- ½ bunch coriander, roughly chopped
- 275g/10oz cod, or other white fish, cubed

Method

Put the garlic, ginger, chilli and tomatoes in blender and blitz until smooth.

Fry the onion in olive oil for 2 minutes, or until translucent, stirring regularly.

Sprinkle in the spices and fry for 30 seconds. Add in the blitzed ingredients and fry for a further 3 minutes.

Add in the coconut oil, coconut milk and salt, then raise the heat to bring to a boil.

Add in the fish and bring to a simmer. Cook for 3 minutes, or until just cooked through.

Stir in the lime juice and most of the coriander, reserving some to garnish.

CHEF'S NOTE

This curry is incredibly quick and versatile to make. Serve on its own as a soup, or with cauliflower rice to soak up the flavoursome juices.

STEAK AND COURGETTI

Ingredients

- 650g /1½lb sirloin steak, sliced into strips
- 4 medium courgettes, spiralized
- 2 tbsp olive oil
- 4 garlic cloves, minced
- 2 tablespoons butter or ghee
- 1 lemon, juice and zest
- 60ml/2floz chicken stock
- ¼ tsp crushed red pepper flakes
- For the marinade:
- 75ml/2½floz soy sauce
- 60ml/2floz lemon juice
- 120ml/4floz olive oil
- 1 tbsp Sriracha sauce

Method

1 Combine the ingredients for the marinade in an airtight container or a Ziploc bag. Add the steak strips into the marinade, seal and allow to marinate in the fridge for at least 30 minutes.

2 Bring the steak to room temperature and heat the oil in a large pan over a medium-high heat — reserve the juices of the marinade for later. Add the steak strips in one layer and season with salt and pepper. Cook for one minute without stirring.

3 Add the minced garlic, then stir the steak for another minute or two to cook the other side. Remove the steak from the pan and set aside.

4 In the same pan, add the butter, lemon juice and zest, red pepper flakes, chicken stock, and remaining marinade juices.

5 Bring to a simmer and allow to reduce for 2-3 minutes, stirring regularly.

6 Add the spiralised courgette and toss for 2-3 minutes. Add the steak strips back to the pan and stir for another minute. Serve immediately.

CHEF'S NOTE

The use of soy in hormone regulating diets has been much debated, but it can raise your oestrogen levels, making it a good choice if you're looking to raise your sex-drive.

ROAST CHICKEN

·············· *Ingredients* ··············

- 1 large chicken
- 1 lemon
- 2 tbsp fresh chopped Italian herbs (basil, oregano & rosemary)

- 2 tbsp butter
- 1 garlic clove, crushed
- Flaky sea salt

·············· *Method* ··············

Preheat the oven to 220C/425F/Gas Mark 7.

Cut the lemon in half and scatter a little salt over the cut side before placing it inside the chicken's cavity

Use a fork to combine the fresh herbs and butter together.

Lift the skin of the bird and use your fingers or the back of a spoon to push the herbed butter right up underneath the skin.

Place it in the oven and cook according to the label instructions (generally this is 20 minutes per lb/450g plus an extra 10-20 minutes at the end).

6 Remove the chicken from the oven, squeeze the juice from the remaining lemon half over the top and sprinkle with salt.

CHEF'S NOTE
Use whichever mix of fresh herbs you prefer and eat the crispy skin to ensure high levels of fat in your diet.

CHICKEN KEBABS

Ingredients

- 3 tbsp natural yoghurt
- 1 tsp garam masala or curry powder
- 1 tsp chilli powder
- 2 tsp lime or lemon juice

- 2 tsp fresh coriander, chopped (optional)
- 1 fresh red chilli, finely chopped
- 750g/1lb 11oz chicken breasts, cubed

Method

1 Mix together the yoghurt, garam masala, chilli powder, lime juice, coriander and red chilli.

2 Marinate the chicken in the yoghurt mixture for an hour or two.

3 Preheat a griddle pan to hot.

4 Thread the chicken onto kebab skewers and cook on the griddle until the chicken is tender and cooked all the way through.

CHEF'S NOTE
It is important that your gut is in good shape so that your body can absorb all of the nutrient-rich food you'll be eating. Yoghurt contains healthy bacteria to balance your gut and, in turn, your hormones.

BEEF & HORSERADISH

Ingredients

- 12 shallots
- 2 tbsp olive oil, plus extra for brushing
- 1 sprig fresh thyme
- 1kg/2¼lb good quality steak
- 2 tbsp fresh horseradish, grated

- 200ml/7floz crème fraîche
- 1 tsp white wine vinegar
- 1 sprig of fresh rosemary
- 1 orange (zest only)

Method

Preheat the oven to 180°C/350°F/Gas Mark 4. Toss the unpeeled shallots in the olive oil, season with sea salt and black pepper, then place in a shallow baking dish with the thyme sprig. Cover tightly with foil and bake in the oven for 45mins, or until soft.

Meanwhile, preheat a heavy griddle pan that's large enough to hold the beef comfortably.

Remove all the fat and any sinew from the beef, season well, and brush with olive oil. Place on the hot griddle for 2-3 mins to sear and brown all over (cook the steak to your liking). Remove from the pan and place on a plate to cool for about 30 mins.

Mix the horseradish into the crème fraîche. Season well with salt, pepper and the vinegar.

5 Finely chop the rosemary and finely grate the zest of the orange.

6 Thinly slice the beef with a sharp carving knife and lay 3 slices on each plate. Peel some of the warm shallots, tear them in half and lay a piece on top of each piece of beef.

7 Spoon a little horseradish crème fraîche on top and sprinkle the plates with the rosemary and orange zest before serving.

STEAK WITH BEARNAISE SAUCE

Ingredients

- 4 steaks of your choice
- 300g/11oz butter
- 4 tbsp white wine vinegar
- 4 shallots, chopped
- 3 tbsp chopped fresh tarragon, plus 2 tbsp

- whole tarragon leaves
- 4 free-range eggs, yolks only
- 1 tsp lemon juice

Method

1 Melt the butter in a small, heavy-based saucepan over a low heat. When the butter is foaming, remove the pan from the heat and leave it to stand for a few minutes so that the white solids sink to the bottom of the pan. Strain the butter through a fine sieve and discard the solids.

2 Pour the vinegar into a small pan. Add the shallots, chopped tarragon and salt, to taste. Heat gently over a medium heat until the liquid has reduced by more than half. Strain and set aside until completely cool.

3 Whilst the liquid cools cook the steaks to your liking and place to one side to rest while you finish making the sauce.

4 Lightly beat the egg yolks with one teaspoon of water. Stir the egg yolk mixture into the cooled vinegar, then add the lemon juice.

5 Pour the mixture into a bowl suspended over a pan of simmering water (do not allow base of the bowl to touch the water). Whisk constantly until the sauce has thickened enough to coat the back of a spoon and has increased in volume.

6 Remove the bowl from the heat and slowly pour in the butter in a steady stream, whisking continuously, until the mixture is thick and smooth Fold in the tarragon leaves and season, to taste, with salt and freshly ground black pepper.

7 Serve the sauce poured over the steaks.

ROSEMARY LAMB

Ingredients

- 1 lamb leg (use organic lamb)
- 5 stalks fresh rosemary, chopped
- 1 tbsp olive oil
- 2 garlic cloves, crushed

Method

Slash the flesh of the leg, rub all of the ingredients all over, making sure you work it into the cuts, and leave to marinate for at least an hour, or preferably overnight.

Preheat the oven to 180C/350F/Gas Mark 4.

Cook the lamb in a roasting tin for around for 25mins per lb/450g + 25 mins at the end. This should mean the lamb is 'medium' cooked.

If you prefer it 'well done' cook for a little longer, although lamb is best served slightly pink.

CHEF'S NOTE
This lamb goes wonderfully with roasted root vegetables for a Sunday lunch to remember, and you can serve any leftovers with the beetroot and feta salad.

LAMB CASSEROLE

Ingredients

- 300g/11oz diced lamb shoulder
- 6 tbsp olive oil
- 4 garlic cloves, crushed
- 1 sprig fresh rosemary
- 2 bay leaves
- 568ml/16floz dry white wine

- ½ lemon, juice only
- 1 onion, sliced
- 1 celery stalk, sliced
- 8 anchovy fillets in oil
- 85g/3oz capers

Method

1 Place the lamb pieces into a large bowl and add three tablespoons of olive oil, the garlic, rosemary, bay leaves, white wine and lemon juice. Stir until well combined, then cover and marinate in the fridge overnight.

2 Preheat the oven to 170C/325F/Gas Mark 3.

3 Remove the lamb pieces from the marinade (but keep the marinade) and pat dry with kitchen paper.

4 Heat the remaining olive oil in a large pan over a medium heat. Add the lamb pieces to the hot oil and fry for 4-5 minutes, or until golden brown all over. Transfer to an ovenproof casserole dish.

5 Pour the reserved marinade into the hot frying pan and warm through, then add it to the casserole dish with the lamb, along with the onion, celery, anchovies and capers. Place in the oven and cook for 1 hr or until the lamb is tender.

CHEF'S NOTE
Fish and meat may seem like an unusual combination, but anchovies make a great match for lamb and are full of omega-3 fatty acids, which have impressive anti-inflammatory properties.

PESTO PORK

Ingredients

- 2 pork steaks
- 2 slices prosciutto
- 100g/3½oz crème fraîche

- 1½ tbsp pesto
- 25g/1oz grated parmesan
- 1 tbsp pine nuts

Method

Heat oven to 200C/400F/Gas Mark 6.

Season the pork all over, then wrap each fillet in a slice of prosciutto. Put into a large baking dish. Dot the crème fraîche and pesto between the steaks and over the exposed ends of the pork. Scatter the cheese over the top.

Bake for 25-30 minutes, adding the pine nuts halfway through, until the crème fraîche has made a sauce around the meat, and the cheese and prosciutto are turning golden.

CHEF'S NOTE

Full of healthy fats, this delicious dish goes well when served with streamed green vegetables or mashed cauliflower. Pine nuts contain vitamins A, B, C, D and E, and lutein.

FISH STEW

Ingredients

- 1 handful flat-leaf parsley leaves, chopped
- 1 garlic clove, finely chopped
- 1 lemon, zest and juice
- 2 tbsp olive oil
- 1 small onion, finely sliced
- 1 tsp paprika
- Pinch cayenne pepper
- 400g/14fl oz tin chopped tomatoes
- 1 fish stock cube
- 100g/3½oz raw peeled king prawns
- 250g/9oz skinless fish fillets, cut into very large chunks

Method

1 In a small bowl, mix the parsley with ½ the garlic and lemon zest, then set aside. Heat 2 tbsp of oil in a large sauté pan. Throw in the onion, cover the pan, then sweat for about 5 minutes, or until the onion has softened. Add the remaining oil, garlic and spices, then cook for a further 2 minutes.

2 Pour over the lemon juice and sizzle for a moment. Add the tomatoes and crumble in the stock. Season with a little salt, then cover the pan. Simmer everything for 15-20 minutes.

3 Stir through the prawns and nestle the fish chunks into the top of the stew. Reduce the heat and recover the pan, then cook for about 8 minutes, stirring very gently once or twice. When the fish is cooked through, remove from the heat, scatter with the parsley mix and serve.

CHEF'S NOTE

This recipe is easy to scale up, or can be adapted to use chicken instead of fish. Use oily fish to ensure you have enough omega 3, as your body cannot make it naturally.

VEGETABLE CURRY

Ingredients

- 1 tbsp coconut oil
- 2 onions, finely chopped
- 250g/9oz chopped vegetables of your choice
- 2 garlic cloves, crushed
- 20g/¾oz ginger, finely grated
- 2 tsp garam masala

- ½ tsp hot chilli powder
- 400g/14oz tin chopped tomatoes
- 600ml/1pt chicken stock
- 100g/3½oz dried red split lentils, drained and rinsed
- 2 bay leaves

To serve:
- 150g/5oz natural yoghurt
- 1 tbsp roughly chopped fresh coriander leaves

Method

Place the coconut oil in a large saucepan over a medium heat. Cook the onions for 5 minutes, stirring regularly, until softened and very lightly browned.

Cut your vegetables into bite size pieces and add to the pan. Cook for 2 minutes, turning occasionally. Stir in the garlic, ginger, garam masala and chilli powder, and cook for a few seconds, stirring constantly.

Tip the tomatoes into the pan and add the chicken stock, lentils and bay leaves. Bring to the boil, then cover loosely with a lid and simmer gently for 35 minutes, or until the vegetables are tender and the lentils have completely broken down. Stir occasionally and remove the lid for the last 10 minutes of cooking time.

4 Season the curry to taste. Serve topped with the yoghurt and sprinkled with coriander.

CHEF'S NOTE
Coconut oil regulates blood sugar and insulin, and boosts thyroid functionality, helping to restore balance to your system.

MEXICAN PULLED PORK

Ingredients

- 1.35kg/3lb boneless pork shoulder
- 2 tsp cumin
- 2 tsp garlic powder
- 2 tsp onion powder
- 2 tsp salt
- 2 tsp paprika
- 2 tbsp hot sauce

Method

1 Add the pork shoulder to a large slow cooker.

2 In a small bowl, stir together the cumin, garlic powder, onion powder, salt, and paprika. Rub the mixture into the pork, making sure to coat all sides.

3 Pour the hot sauce into the bottom of the slow cooker.

4 Cook on low for 8 hours, or high for 4 hours. The pork is ready when it easily shreds with a fork.

5 Shred the pork and stir the meat into the juices in the bottom of the slow cooker.

CHEF'S NOTE

This delicious meat contains none of the sugar that BBQ pulled pork has. Serve 'fajita-style', in lettuce wraps with guacamole and salsa, for plenty of healthy hormone-balancing fats.

MOULES MARINIÈRE

Ingredients

- 1.75kg/4lb mussels
- 1 garlic clove, finely chopped
- 2 shallots, finely chopped
- 1 tbsp butter
- 1 bouquet garni of parsley, thyme and bay leaves
- 100ml/3½floz dry white wine
- 120ml/4floz double cream
- 1 handful of parsley leaves, coarsely chopped

Method

Wash the mussels under plenty of cold, running water. Discard any open ones that won't close when lightly squeezed.

Pull out the tough, fibrous beards protruding from between the tightly closed shells and then knock off any barnacles with a large knife. Give the mussels another quick rinse to remove any little pieces of shell.

Soften the garlic and shallots in the butter with the bouquet garni in a large pan, big enough to take all the mussels - it should only be half full.

Add the mussels and wine, turn up the heat, then cover and steam them open in their own juices for 3-4 minutes. Give the pan a good shake every now and then.

5 Remove the bouquet garni, add the cream and chopped parsley, then remove from the heat.

6 Spoon into four large warmed bowls and serve, discarding any mussels which have not opened during cooking.

CHEF'S NOTE

Seafood is a fantastic source of protein, but those wishing to balance their hormones should be wary of mercury which is an endocrine disruptor. Mussels however are generally a safe source.

KETO PIZZA

Ingredients

For the base:
- 150g/5oz mozzarella cheese, shredded
- 100g/3½oz almond flour
- 2 tbsp cream cheese
- 1 tsp white wine vinegar
- 1 egg
- ½ tsp salt

For the topping:
- 6 cherry tomatoes, halved
- 1 tbsp butter
- 120ml/4floz unsweetened tomato sauce
- ½ tsp dried oregano
- 125g/4oz mozzarella cheese, shredded
- 6 torn basil leaves

Method

1 Preheat the oven to 200C/400F/Gas Mark 6.

2 To make the base, heat the mozzarella and cream cheese in a small, non-stick pan on medium heat, or in a bowl in the microwave oven. Stir until they melt together. Add the other ingredients and mix well.

3 Moisten your hands with olive oil and flatten the dough on parchment paper, making a circle about 8 inches (20 cm) in diameter. You can also use a rolling pin to flatten the dough between two sheets of parchment paper.

4 Remove top parchment sheet (if used). Prick the crust all over with a fork and bake in the oven for 10–12 mins until golden brown. Remove from the oven.

5 Spread a thin layer of tomato sauce on the crust. Top with the tomatoes and plenty of cheese. Bake for 10–15 minutes, or until the cheese has melted. Top with the basil leaves and serve.

CHEF'S NOTE

Pizza may seem a no-go when you're following a ketogenetic diet, but using alternatives like almond flour means that you can still enjoy your favourite foods.

SERVES 6

RUSTIC BOLOGNAISE

Ingredients

- 700g/1lb 9oz stewing steak
- 5 tbsp vegetable oil
- 4 rashers smoked streaky bacon or pancetta, cut into 1cm slices
- 1 large onion, finely chopped
- 4 garlic cloves, crushed

- 75g/3oz pitted black olives, drained and rinsed
- 600ml/1pt red wine
- 1 400g/14oz can chopped tomatoes
- 2 tbsp tomato puree

- 600ml/1pt beef stock
- 2 large bay leaves
- 3 sprigs thyme
- 1 rosemary stalk, about 12cm long, leaves finely chopped

Method

Season the beef well with salt and pepper.

Heat 2 tablespoons of the oil in a large frying pan.

Fry the chunks of beef over a medium-high heat until browned on all sides, turning every now and then. This may take a few batches. As the meat is browned, transfer it to a large flameproof casserole dish, or saucepan with a lid.

Add a little more oil to the pan in which you browned the meat and fry the bacon for 2–3 minutes, or until brown and crispy, then scatter it over the meat.

Fry the chopped onion, in the same pan as before, over a low heat for 5 minutes, stirring often. Stir in the garlic, olives and cook for a further 2 minutes, stirring occasionally.

6 Add the onions to the meat in the casserole dish, then pour in the wine. Stir in the tomatoes, tomato puree and beef stock. Add all the herbs and bring the mixture to a simmer.

7 Stir well and cover the casserole loosely with a lid, then turn the heat down low and leave to simmer very gently for 2½ hours, or until the meat is completely tender and falling apart.

8 Remove the lid every now and then and stir. If the liquid reduces too much, add a little extra water. The sauce should be fairly thick at the end of the cooking time. Remove the thyme and rosemary stalks, and the bay leaves, then season to taste.

9 Serve with freshly grated Parmesan.

MACKEREL WITH ROAST TOMATOES

Ingredients

- 375g/13oz mixed red and yellow cherry tomatoes
- 320g/11½oz fine green beans, trimmed
- 2 garlic cloves, finely chopped
- 2 tbsp lemon juice
- 8 mackerel fillets
- 1 lemon, rind only, finely grated
- 2 tsp baby capers, drained
- 2 spring onions, finely sliced
- 1 tsp olive oil

Method

1 Preheat the oven to 200C/400F Fan/Gas Mark 6.

2 Put the tomatoes in an ovenproof dish with the beans, garlic and lemon juice, then drizzle over the oil. Season with salt and freshly ground black pepper and mix well. Bake for 10 minutes, or until the tomatoes and beans are tender.

3 Meanwhile, tear off 4 large sheets of foil and line with non-stick baking paper. Place 2 fish fillets on each piece of baking paper, then scatter over the lemon rind, capers and spring onions, and season with salt and freshly ground black pepper. Fold over the paper-lined foil and scrunch the edges together to seal. Place the parcels on a large baking tray.

4 Place the fish parcels next to the vegetables in the oven and bake for 8-10 minutes, or until the flesh flakes easily when pressed in the centre with a knife. Spoon the vegetables on to four serving plates, top each with two fish fillets and serve.

CHEF'S NOTE

Mackerel contains a good amount of selenium and a small quantity of iodine, so they are a thyroid-supportive food, perfect for those looking to balance their hormones.

SNACKS
SWEET TREATS
& SIDE DISHES

CRANBERRY 'RICE'

Ingredients

- 175g/6oz pecans
- 2 tbsp butter
- 1 shallot, thinly sliced
- 250ml/8½fl oz chicken stock
- 1½kg/3lb6oz riced cauliflower
- 2 sprigs fresh thyme

- 1 bay leaf
- 1 tsp sea salt
- ½ tsp ground black pepper
- 2 tbsp chopped fresh flat-leaf parsley
- 125g/4oz grated Parmesan cheese
- 60g/2½oz sugar free dried cranberries

Method

1 Preheat the oven to 180C/350F/Gas Mark 4. Spread the pecans in a single layer on a rimmed baking sheet and roast for 8 minutes.

2 Meanwhile, heat the butter in a large frying pan over a medium heat. Add the shallot and sauté until it is soft and translucent.

3 Add the stock to the pan and, using a rubber spatula, scrape and mix in any bits that are stuck to the bottom of the pan.

4 Add the riced cauliflower, thyme, bay leaf, salt, and pepper to the pan. Cook for about 15 minutes, or until all of the liquid has evaporated, and the cauliflower is completely cooked and tender.

5 Remove the thyme sprigs and bay leaf and discard. Mix in the roasted pecans, Parmesan cheese, and dried cranberries. Taste and add mo salt and pepper, if desired.

CHEF'S NOTE
Eating too much fruit isn't wise when you're trying to control your insulin levels, but cranberries are rich in anti-oxidants and alkaline, making them a good choice for when you do indulge.

BABA GANOUSH

Ingredients

- 3 aubergines
- 3 garlic cloves, crushed with a teaspoon of salt
- 1 lemon, juice only

- 2 tbsp tahini
- 3 tbsp olive oil
- 1 tbsp chopped flat leaf parsley

Method

Prick the aubergines with a fork, then grill until the skin is charred and blackened, and the flesh feels soft when you press it (this will take approximately 15-20 minutes - turn halfway through cooking).

In a pestle and mortar, crush the garlic with the lemon juice, tahini, olive oil and pepper.

When cool enough to handle, cut the aubergines in half and scoop out the flesh. Mix the soft flesh with the remaining ingredients.

Place in a serving dish, finish with a drizzle of olive oil and sprinkle the parsley over the top.

CHEF'S NOTE

Tahini is made from ground sesame, a great source of omega-6. There is some evidence that they may be able to help bind excess hormone metabolites and increase their clearance from the body.

BEETROOT TZATZIKI

Ingredients

- 1 cooked beetroot, peeled
- 500g/1lb 2oz plain Greek-style yoghurt
- 1 lemon, juice only
- 1 handful fresh dill
- 2 tbsp fresh mint leaves, chopped
- 2 tbsp cucumber, finely chopped

Method

1 Put the beetroot into a food processor and blend until finely chopped.

2 Transfer to a bowl and mix in all the remaining ingredients.

3 Season with salt and black pepper.

4 Serve with crudités for dipping.

CHEF'S NOTE
Beetroot supports the liver and is rich in iron, B vitamins, potassium, magnesium, and folate. They help usher toxins (like excess oestrogen) out of the liver.

CELERIAC REMOULADE

Ingredients

- ½ small celeriac, cut into thin strips
- ½ lemon, juice only
- 2 tbsp double cream
- 3 tbsp good-quality mayonnaise
- 2 tsp Dijon mustard

Method

Place the celeriac strips into a bowl, along with the lemon juice, and stir to combine.

Mix the double cream, mayonnaise and mustard together, then stir into the celeriac.

Season with salt and white pepper.

Place in the fridge for a couple of hours to allow the flavours to develop before serving.

CHEF'S NOTE

Celeriac is a really useful low-carb vegetable when you're following a ketogenic diet. It's delicious raw but also cooks well to make mash, rostis or even chips!

MAYONNAISE

Ingredients

- 300ml/10½floz groundnut oil
- 2 eggs, yolks only
- 1 garlic clove, crushed
- 1 tsp mustard powder

- 1 level tsp salt
- Freshly milled black pepper
- 1 tsp white wine vinegar

Method

1 Place the egg yolks into a bowl, add the crushed garlic, mustard powder, salt and a little freshly milled black pepper. Mix together well. Then, holding the groundnut oil in a jug in one hand and an electric hand whisk in the other, add a drop of oil to the egg mixture and whisk this in.

2 Add the oil drop by drop until mixture thickens and becomes very stiff and lumpy. Then add a teaspoon of vinegar, which will thin the mixture down.

3 Begin pouring the oil in a very, very thin but steady stream, keeping the beaters going all the time. When all the oil has been added, taste and add more salt and pepper if desired.

CHEF'S NOTE

Mayonnaise is something you're likely to eat lots of on a ketogenic diet, as it's a delicious way of adding fat to your food. Rather than bottled, which can contain sugar, try making your own.

MACKEREL PÂTÉ

Ingredients

- 2 smoked mackerel, skinned and boned
- 125g/4oz cottage cheese
- 150g/5oz sour cream
- ½ lemon, juice only
- Pinch grated nutmeg
- Pinch cayenne pepper
- 2 lemons cut into wedges

Method

Blend all the ingredients.

Season to taste with the cayenne pepper, nutmeg and salt.

Put into individual dishes or one large one.

Cover with clingfilm and chill for at least two hours.

Sprinkle with a little cayenne and serve with lemon wedges.

CHEF'S NOTE

This pâté is a great way to ensure you getting plenty of oily fish in your diet. It also works well with smoked trout or hot smoked salmon.

SATAY CHICKEN WRAPS

Ingredients

- 1 iceberg lettuce
- 1 large chicken breast, cooked
- ⅓ cucumber
- 1 carrot, peeled and cut into fine matchsticks
- ½ red pepper, deseeded and cut into fine matchsticks
- 5 radishes, trimmed and thinly sliced
- 1 small bunch fresh coriander leaves
- 1 long red chilli, finely chopped
- 3 spring onions, finely sliced
- Lime wedges, for squeezing
- For the satay sauce:
- 3 tbsp crunchy peanut butter
- 1 tbsp chilli sauce
- 2 tsp dark soy sauce
- 2 tsp fresh lime juice

Method

1 To make the satay sauce, put the peanut butter in a small bowl and stir in 2 tablespoons of just-boiled water. Mix in the chilli sauce, soy sauce and lime juice. Transfer to a shallow serving dish and place in the centre of a large board or platter.

2 Trim the bottom of the lettuce and carefully separate 8 large leaves.

3 Cut the chicken breast into thin slices and place on the board or platter with the satay sauce. Arrange the lettuce leaves, cucumber, carrot, pepper, radishes and coriander in separate piles beside the chicken. Put the chilli and spring onions in separate small dishes on the board.

4 To assemble the wraps, place a selection of the vegetables into the lettuce leaves. Add a couple of chicken slices and then top with the satay sauce, spring onions and chillies to taste. Garnish with the fresh coriander and add a squeeze of lime, before wrapping the rest of the leaf around the filling. Serve immediately.

CHEF'S NOTE

These wraps are a fun way to dine with a group, plus there are plenty of alkaline and antioxidant rich vegetables, as well as healthy fat from the peanut butter.

TAPENADE

Ingredients

- 1 garlic clove, crushed
- 1 lemon, juice only
- 3 tbsp capers, chopped
- 6 anchovy fillets, chopped

- 250g/9oz black olives, pitted
- 1 small bunch fresh parsley, chopped
- 2-4 tbsp extra virgin olive oil

Method

Mix all the ingredients together, adding enough olive oil to form a paste.

Alternatively, for a smoother texture, add the garlic, lemon juice, capers and anchovy into a food processor and blitz for about 10 seconds.

Add the olives and parsley and enough olive oil to make a paste.

Season to taste.

CHEF'S NOTE

Olives and olive oil are good additions to your diet, as they may help to balance levels of a hormone that regulates the appetite and stimulates the digestion of fat and protein.

CHILLI KALE

Ingredients

- 3 tbsp extra virgin olive oil
- 1 large onion, sliced
- 2 sprigs fresh rosemary
- 1 medium or hot fresh red chilli, deseeded and thinly sliced

- 4 garlic cloves, sliced
- 250g/9oz curly kale or cavolo nero, trimmed of tough stems, rinsed and cut into 1cm/½in thick slices

Method

1 Heat the olive oil in a deep, heavy-bottomed lidded pan over a medium heat. Add the onion, turn down the heat and fry gently until very tender.

2 Add the rosemary, chilli and garlic and fry for another minute.

3 Add the kale or cavolo nero and season with salt. Cover with a tight-fitting lid, reduce the heat to its absolute minimum and leave to cook gently for about 20 minutes. Stir once, after five minutes, then again ten minutes later.

4 Remove the rosemary stalks, then taste and adjust the seasoning. Serve immediately.

CHEF'S NOTE

This is a fantastic side dish that's bursting with healthy vegetables, herbs and spices. It would go wonderfully with roast chicken.

AVOCADO FRIES

Ingredients

- 3 avocados
- 1 egg
- 350g/12oz ground almonds

- Aprox. 400ml/14floz sunflower oil
- ¼ tsp cayenne pepper
- ½ tsp salt

Method

Break an egg into a bowl and beat it.

In another bowl, mix the almonds with some salt and cayenne pepper.

Slice each avocado in half and take out the stone. Peel off the skin and slice vertically into 4 or 5 pieces.

Heat a deep fat fryer (or deep pan with lots of oil) to about 180C/350F.

Coat each slice of avocado in the egg. Roll each coated slice in the almond mix until well coated.

Carefully lower each avocado slice into the deep fryer (or pan) and allow each piece to fry for 45-60 seconds, until they turn a light brown.

7 Transfer quickly to a plate lined with a paper towel to soak up the excess oil and east straight away.

CHEF'S NOTE

An unusual treat that's full of healthy fats - they're delicious on the side of some grilled salmon, or simply served with mayonnaise for a TV snack!

SMOKED SALMON FILLED AVOCADO

Ingredients

- 2 avocados
- 175g/6oz smoked salmon
- 175ml/6fl oz crème fraîche, sour cream or mayonnaise
- 2 tbsp lemon juice (optional)

Method

1 Cut the avocados in half and remove the pit.

2 Place a dollop of the crème fraîche, sour cream or mayonnaise in the hollow of the avocado and add the smoked salmon on top.

3 Season to taste with salt, pepper and a squeeze lemon juice before serving.

CHEF'S NOTE

Full of healthy fats, this works as a great starter for a dinner party, or even a healthy breakfast. It also works well with other fatty fish such as smoked mackerel or trout.

GUACAMOLE

Ingredients

- 2 ripe avocados
- 1 garlic clove
- ½ lime, juice only
- 3 tbsp olive oil

- ½ white onion
- 1 small bunch fresh coriander
- 1 tomato, diced

Method

Peel the avocados and mash with a fork.

Grate or chop the onion finely and add to the avocado.

Squeeze the lime and add the juice to the avocado mix.

Add the tomato, olive oil and finely chopped coriander.

Season with salt and pepper and mix well.

CHEF'S NOTE

This Mexican staple is a versatile addition to a keto-alkaline diet. Try it with the Mexican pulled pork in lettuce wraps.

SPICED PECANS AND ALMONDS

Ingredients

- 1 egg white
- 1 tsp cayenne
- 1 tsp cumin
- ½ tsp salt
- 85g/3¼oz each pecans and almonds

Method

1 Heat oven to 150C/300F /Gas Mark 2.

2 Lightly whisk the egg white, then add the spices and salt.

3 Add the pecans and almonds and coat well.

4 Spread out in a single layer on a lightly oiled baking sheet and bake for 12 mins.

5 Cool before eating.

CHEF'S NOTE
Nuts are a great source of protein and healthy fats. Pecans are an excellent source of vitamin E and a rich source of phytosterols, specifically beta-carotene and zeaxanthin.

PEANUT BUTTER

Ingredients

- 300g/11oz peanuts
- 1 tbsp butter

Method

Heat oven to 190C/375F/Gas Mark 5. Spread the peanuts on a baking tray and roast for 10 minutes.

Remove and allow to cool.

Put the roasted peanuts into a food processor with the butter and blitz until you have the type of peanut butter consistency you prefer.

Stop the blender every so often to scrape the sides down, and add a little water to combine, if necessary.

CHEF'S NOTE
Making your own peanut butter ensures that there's no hidden sugars. Try having some spread on your breakfast loaf, or use it to make satay sauce.

CHEESE BITES

······· *Ingredients* ·······

- 150g/5oz cream cheese
- 1 tsp garlic, minced
- 6 olives, chopped

- ¼ tsp Salt
- 2 tbsp Parmesan cheese

······· *Method* ·······

1 In a medium-sized mixing bowl, add the cream cheese, garlic, chopped olives, and salt. Mix until well combined.

2 Scoop into 6 small balls, and place in the fridge to harden slightly before rolling.

3 Pour the parmesan cheese on to a plate, and roll the cream cheese balls in the mixture until completely covered.

4 Store in the fridge until consuming.

CHEF'S NOTE
These cheese balls are a good way of ensuring that you're consuming enough fat, and are a tasty mid-afternoon snack. Try substituting come chopped jalapeños for the olives.

CUCUMBER BITES

Ingredients

- 225g/8oz cream cheese, softened
- 1 tbsp green pepper, finely chopped
- 1 tbsp onion, finely chopped
- 1 tbsp chives, finely chopped
- 2 cucumbers

Method

In a mixing bowl, combine the cream cheese, pepper, chives, and onion. Mix well and set aside.

Cut the cucumbers lengthwise, remove the seeds and fill each cucumber half with the cheese mixture.

Slice the filled cucumber into 1" chunks to serve.

CHEF'S NOTE

These bites make a great snack or canape, but you could also try using the same method of scooping out a cucumber and filling it with your favourite meats or cheeses for a carb-free sandwich!

KETO ICE LOLLIES

Ingredients

- 2 medium avocados
- 2 tbsp lemon juice
- 6 tbsp sweetener

- 250ml/8½fl oz unsweetened almond milk
- 80g/3oz dark chocolate
- 2 tsp cacao butter

Method

1 Place the avocado flesh, lemon juice, almond milk and sweetener into a food processor and combine.

2 Fill 6 lollypop moulds with the mixture and place them into the freezer.

3 Meanwhile, melt the chocolate and cacao butter together over a double boiler.

4 Once the Ice pops are frozen, dip each one into the cooled chocolate.

5 Eat immediately, or place it back into the freezer for later.

CHEF'S NOTE

Dairy can have a negative effect on balancing hormones, so it's a good idea to limit your consumption. Nut milks, like this almond milk, are a great alternative.

AZTEC ICE CREAM

Ingredients

- 1 x 225g/8oz tin full fat coconut milk
- 75g/3oz sweetener
- 80g/3oz dark chocolate
- 1 tsp vanilla extract

- 2 medium avocados
- 1½ tsp ground cinnamon
- ¼ - ¾ tsp chipotle powder

Method

In a medium saucepan over medium heat, whisk the sweetener into the coconut milk until it dissolves. Bring to a simmer.

Remove from heat and add the chopped chocolate. Allow to sit for around 4 minutes, until the chocolate is melted, then whisk until smooth. Whisk in the vanilla extract.

In a blender or food processor, combine the avocado flesh, chocolate mixture, cinnamon, and chipotle. Puree until smooth. Refrigerate until cool, for at least 2 hours.

Transfer the mixture to an ice cream maker and churn until the consistency resembles soft serve ice cream.

5 This can be eaten as a soft serve or transfer to an airtight container and frozen for another few hours if you prefer a firmer consistency.

CHEF'S NOTE

Dark chocolate can aid hormonal balance thanks to its high levels of magnesium and iron, and ability to lower cortisol and boost mood-impacting hormones, serotonin and dopamine.

CHOCOLATE NUT CLUSTERS

Ingredients

- 250g/9oz sugar free dark chocolate chips
- 60ml/2floz coconut oil
- 450g/1lb unsweetened salted mixed nuts

Method

1 Line a rimmed baking sheet or silicone baking mat with parchment paper.

2 In a microwave-safe bowl, combine the chocolate chips with the coconut oil and microwave until melted. Use a rubber spatula to mix until smooth. Allow to cool slightly.

3 Combine the nuts and chocolate, and stir until well coated.

4 Drop large scoops of the mixture onto the prepared baking sheet. Be sure to space them out so they don't run together.

5 Refrigerate until solid. Leftovers can be stored in an airtight container in the fridge for up to 1 week.

CHEF'S NOTE
All nuts (including coconuts) are good sources of mono and polyunsaturated fatty acids (healthy fats) and help balance insulin levels. Experiment with your favourites!

Printed in Great Britain
by Amazon

64307992R00056